Dental Assisting: Tray Setup Guide

Dr. Kimberly Harper, DDS

Copyright © 2018 by Doctor Kimberly Harper Published by DrKimberlyHarper.com The Dental Assisting Academy PO Box 789526 Dallas, Texas 72369 www.thedentalassistignacademy.com

ISBN: 9781794395695

This book contains material protected under international and federal copyright laws and treaties. Any unauthorized reprint or use of this material is prohibited. No part of this book may be reproduced or transmitted in any form or by any means, electronic or mechanical, including photocopying, recording, or by any information storage and retrieval system without express written permission from the publisher except in the case of brief quotations embodied in critical articles and reviews. Limit of Liability / Disclaimer of Warranty: While the publisher and author have used their best efforts in preparing this book, they make no representations or warranties with the respect to the accuracy or completeness of the contents of this book and specifically disclaim any implied warranties of fitness for a particular purpose. No warranty may be created or extended by sales representatives or written sales materials. The advice and strategies contained herein may not be suitable for your situation. You should consult with a doctor where appropriate. Neither the publisher nor author shall be liable for any loss or damages including but not limited to special, incidental, consequential or other damages. Doctor Kimberly Harper's books and products are available through online book retailers. To contact DrKimberlyHarper.com directly, call our Customer Service Department within the U.S. at (800) 888-8978.

This book is dedicated to all of the amazing dental assistants in our dental community. I hope this book is a tool to help you succeed in the awesome career you have chosen. Thank you to the dental assistants that help me create this guide!

Dr. Kimberly

Table of Contents

Introduction 5

Exam 6

Hygiene 7

Composite Fillings 8

Matrix System 10

Crown 11

Crown Seat 13

Extraction 15

Sample Treatment Kit (Instruments) 17

Oral Surgery Instruments (Review) 18

Ways To Advance Your Career 20

5 Ways to Comfort Your Patients 22

Thank You 24

About the Author 25

Introduction

Congratulations on your new career! Welcome to the world of dental assisting. As a dental assistant you have many duties in the office. You are responsible for keeping things flowing in the office and keeping the patients happy.

This tray set up guide was developed to help you be the best dental assistant you can be. Please keep in mind each dentist is different and may prefer different materials, instruments or work sequence. Regardless of the materials or instruments used, I hope this guide is helpful to you.

EXAM

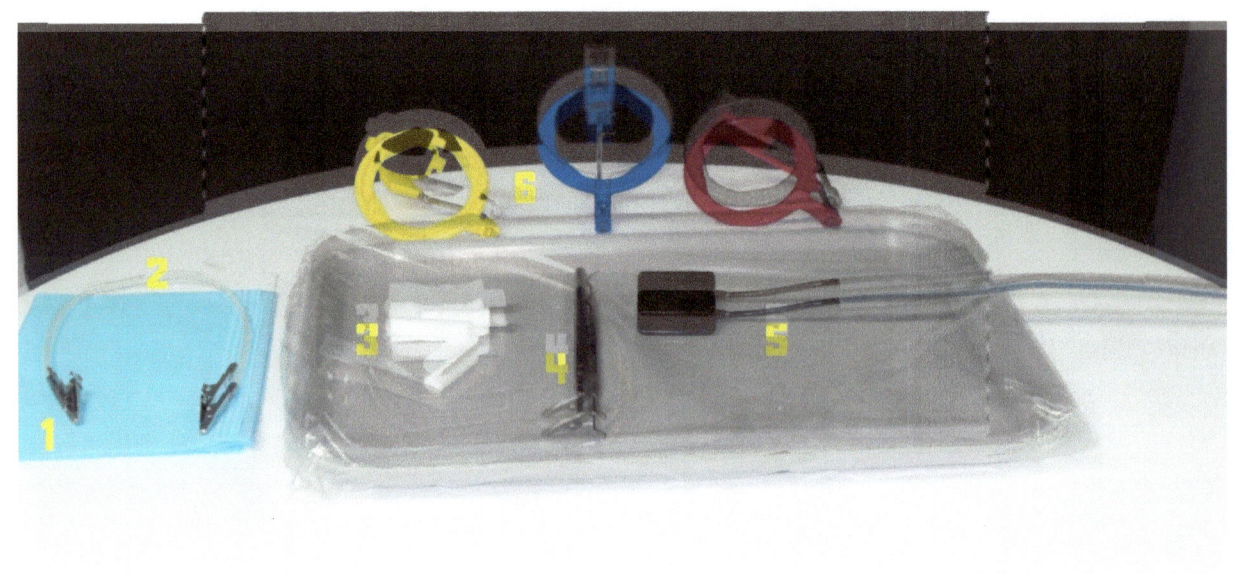

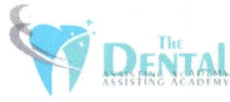

Purpose: An exam tray can be used for a new patient exam, emergency exam, or a consultation.

An exam tray set up consists of the following items:

1. Patient Bib
2. Bib Clip
3. Gauze and Cotton Rolls (2-4 pieces)
4. Basic Instrument Kit (Mouth Mirror & Explorer)
5. Digital X-ray Sensor
6. X-ray Holders
   Yellow: Posterior PA X-rays
   Blue: Anterior PA X-rays
   Red: Bitewing X-rays

Hygiene

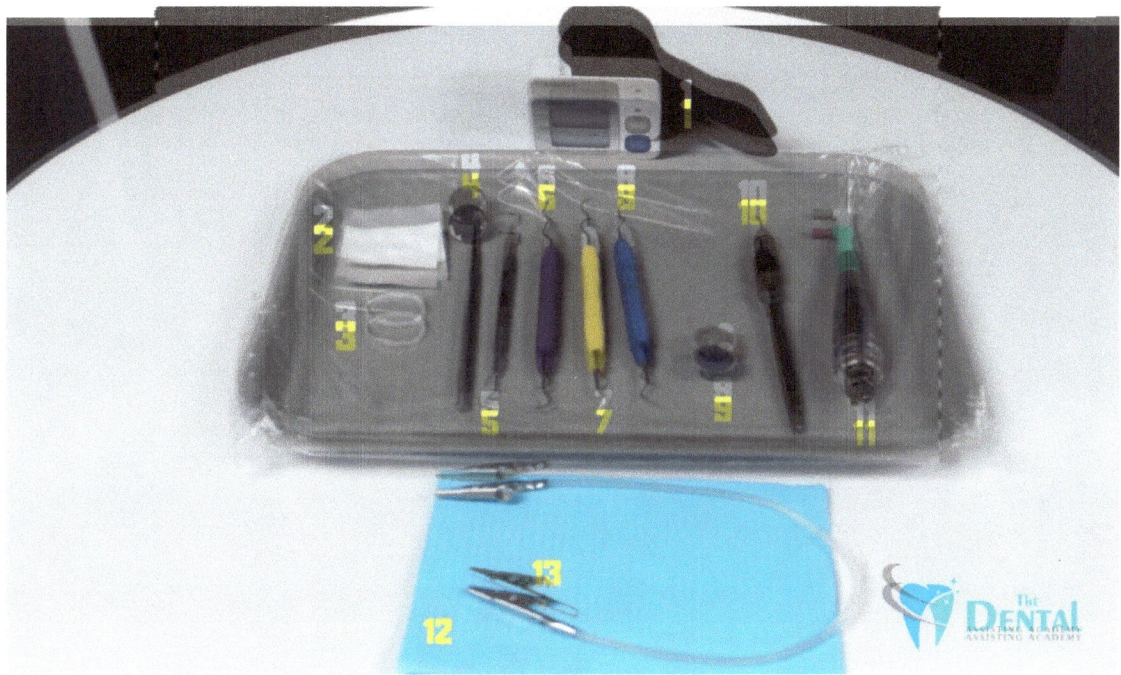

Purpose: A hygiene tray can be used for a basic adult or child cleaning and scaling and root planning (SRP). Additional supplies may be needed for SRP.

The tray set up consists of the following items:

1. Wrist Blood Pressure Cuff
2. Gauze
3. Floss
4. Mirror
5. Periodontal Probe and Explorer
6. Hygiene Scaler
7. Hygiene Scaler
8. Hygiene Scaler
9. Prophy Paste
10. Cavitron Tip
11. Prophy Handpiece
12. Patient Bib
13. Bib Clip

Composite Fillings

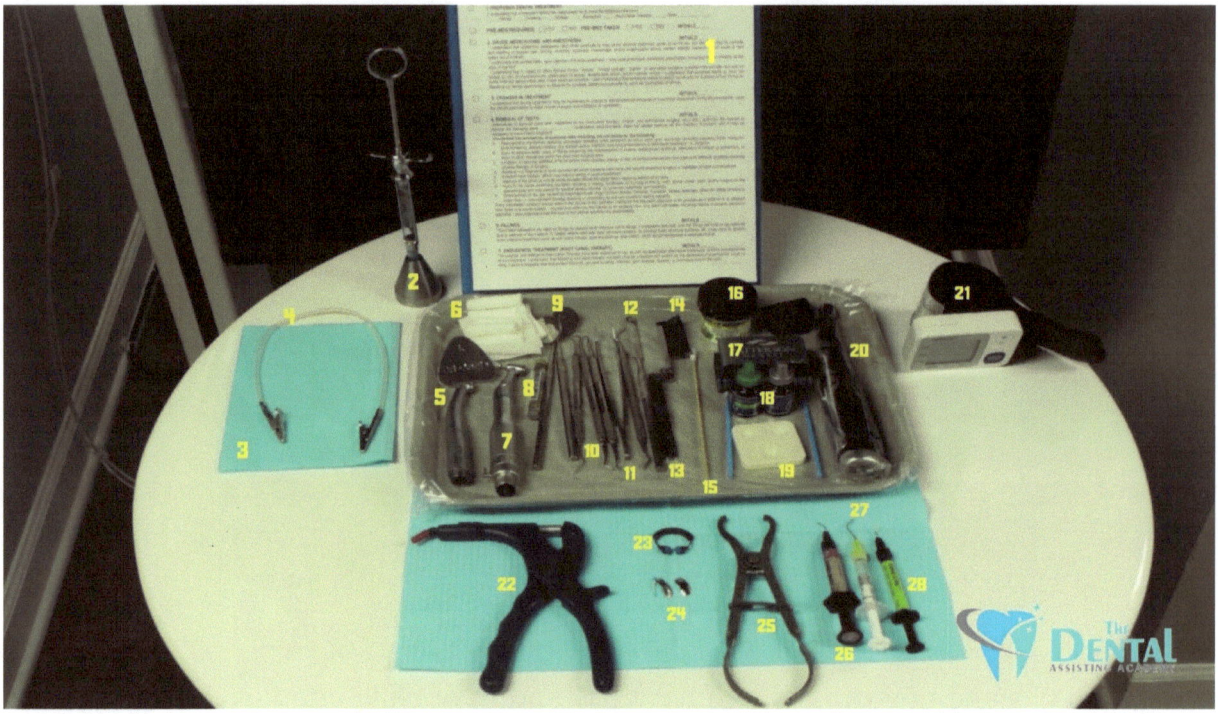

Purpose: This tray set up can be used for composite or amalgam fillings.

The tray set up includes the following items:

1. Consent Form
2. Syringe and needle (Short or long gauge depends on dentist's preference)
3. Patient Bib
4. Bib Clip
5. High Speed Handpiece
6. Cotton Rolls, Gauze, Dry Angles
7. Slow Speed Handpiece
8. Anesthetic Carpule
9. Instrument Pack
10. Instrument Pack
11. Instrument Pack
12. Instrument Pack
13. Instrument Pack

14. Instrument Pack
15. Cotton Tip Applicator
16. Topical Gel
17. Bur Block
18. Bond
19. Well or Dappen Dish for Bond
20. Curing Light
21. Wrist Blood Pressure Cuff
22. Composite Gun
23. Matrix Ring
24. Sectional Matrix Band
25. Ring Placement Forceps
26. Flowable Composite
27. Hemostatic Agent (Viscostat)
28. Base Liner (Limelight)

Matrix System

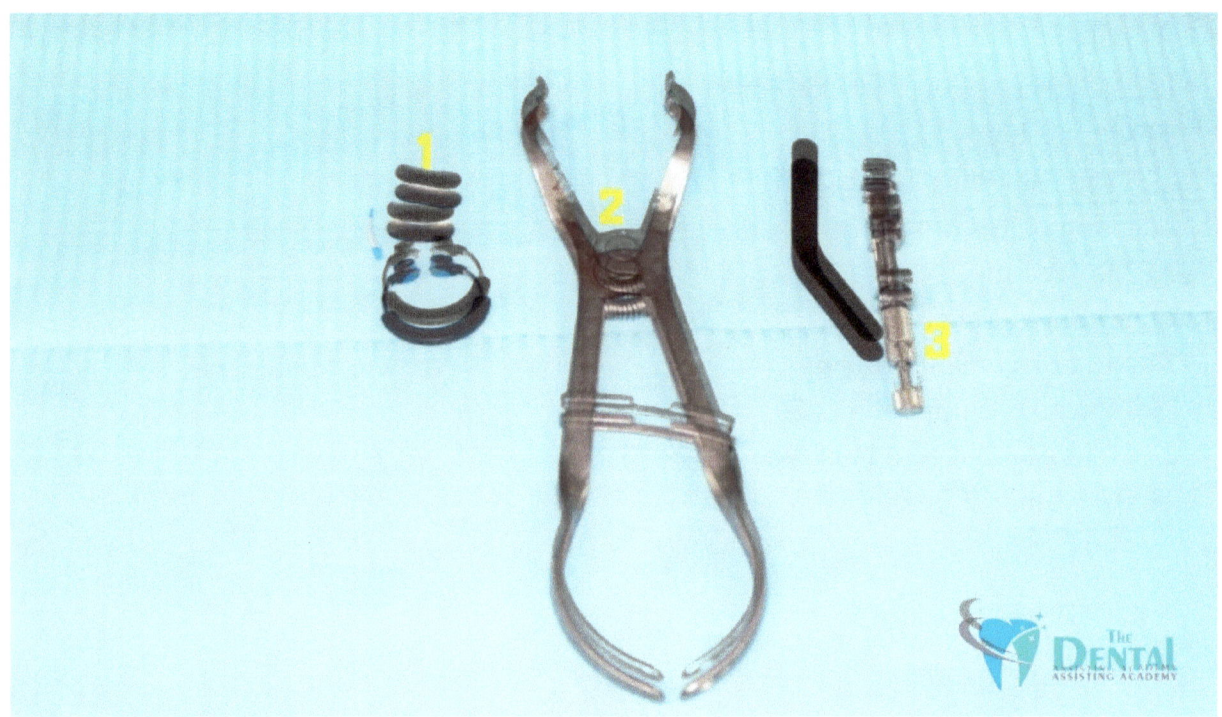

Purpose: A matrix band is used for interproximal fillings (i.e. MO, DO, MOD)

1. Sectional Matrix Band System – ring, wedge and sectional bands
2. Ring Placement Forceps
3. Tofflemire System – tofflemire holder and band

CROWN

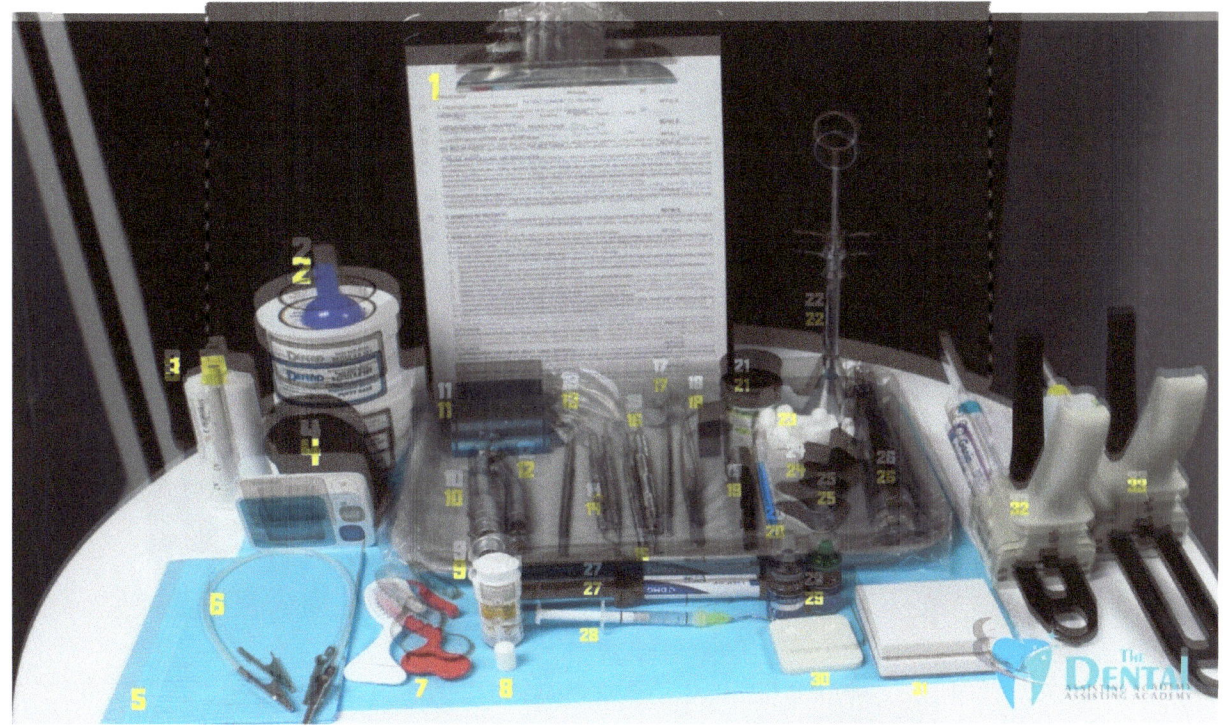

Purpose: This tray set up can be used for crown preparation, onlays and inlays and veneers.

This tray set up includes the following items:

1. Consent Form
2. Putty Material for Preliminary Impression
3. Temporary Crown Material
4. Wrist Blood Pressure Cuff
5. Patient Bib
6. Bib Clip
7. Impression trays – Quadrant tray (White for preliminary, Red for Final)
8. Impression Cap
9. Retraction Cord
10. Slow Speed Handpiece
11. Bur Block
12. High Speed Handpiece
13. Instrument Pack

14. Instrument Pack
15. Instrument Pack
16. Instrument Pack
17. Instrument Pack
18. Instrument Pack
19. Instrument Pack
20. Instrument Pack
21. Topical Gel
22. Syringe and Needle (Short or Long Gauge depending on dentist's preference)
23. Cotton Rolls & Gauze
24. Bite Block
25. Dri-Angle
26. Curing Light
27. Build Up Material (Luxacore)
28. Hemostatic Agent (Viscostat)
29. Bond
30. Well or Dappen Dish for Bond
31. Mixing Pad
32. Heavy Body Impression Material in Impression Gun
33. Light Body Impression Material in Impression Gun

Crown Seat

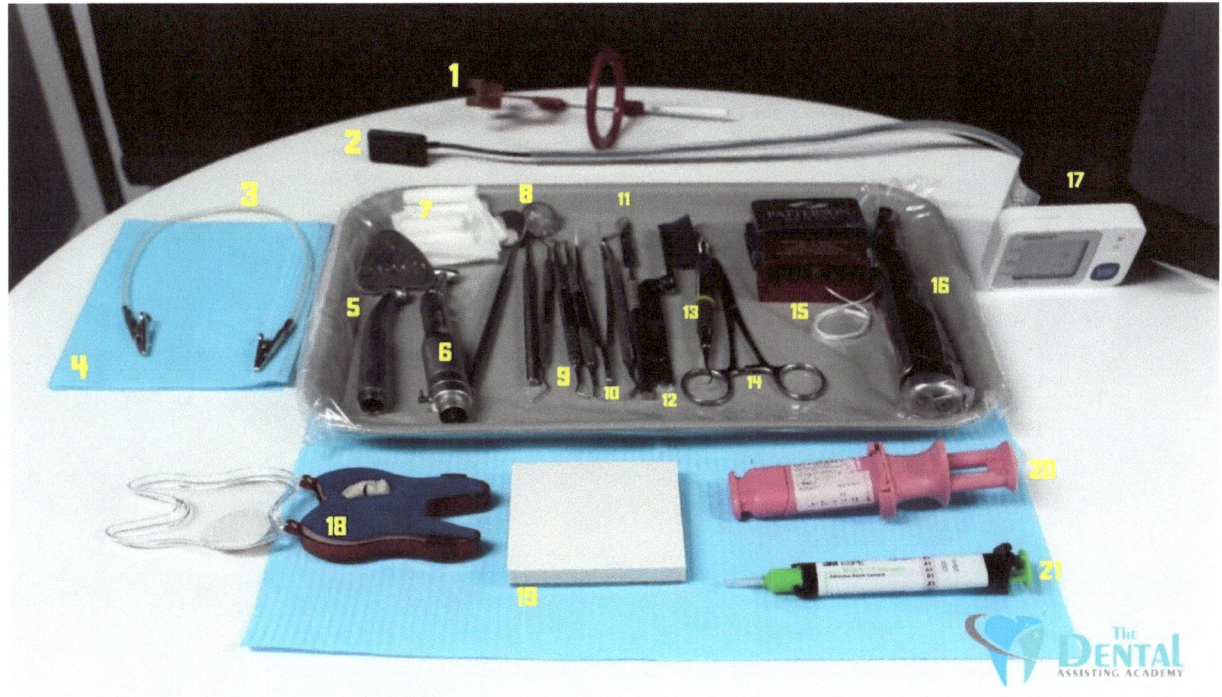

1. X-ray Holder – Bite-Wing
2. Digital X-ray Sensor
3. Bib Clip
4. Patient Bib
5. High Speed Handpiece
6. Slow Speed Handpiece
7. Cotton Rolls and Gauze
8. Instrument Pack
9. Instrument Pack
10. Instrument Pack
11. Instrument Pack
12. Instrument Pack
13. Scaler
14. Hemostat
15. Bur Block
16. Curing Light

17. Wrist Blood Pressure Cuff
18. Crown
19. Mixing Pad
20. Cement – Fuji Cem (PFM or Metal Restorations)
21. Cement – Rely X Ultimate (Ceramic Restorations)

EXTRACTION

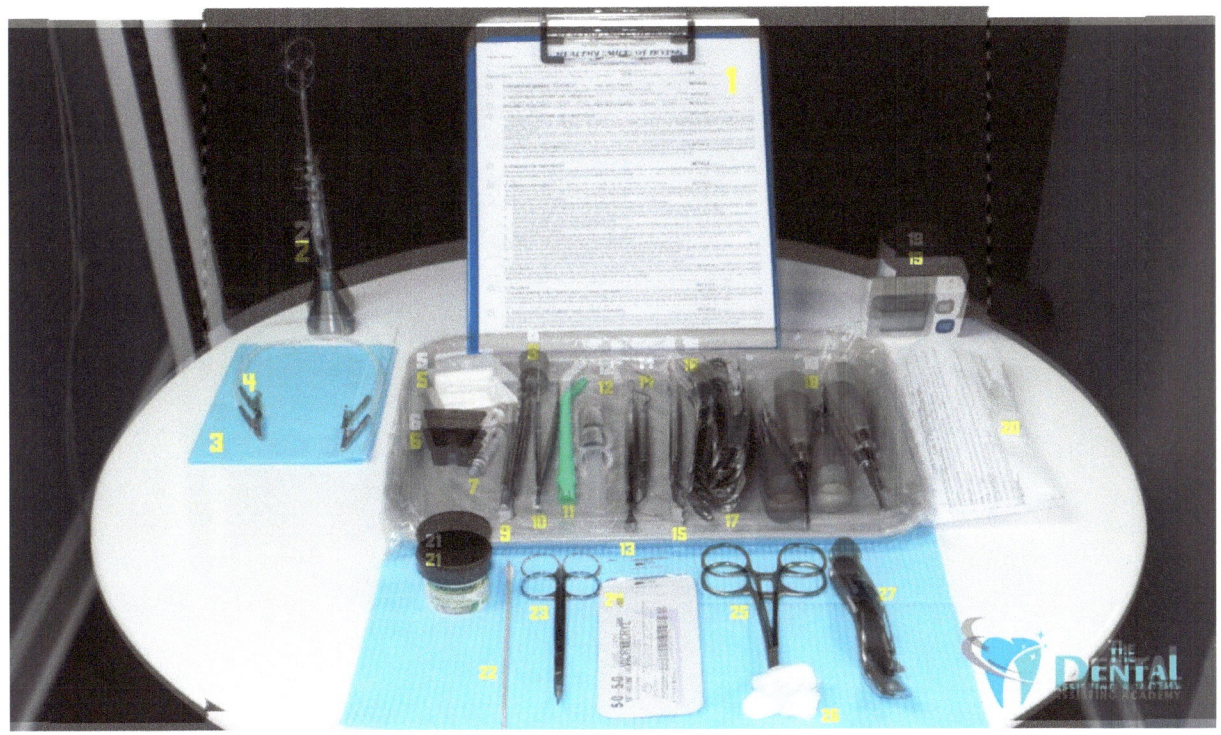

1. Consent Form
2. Syringe and Needle (Short or Long Gauge depending on dentist's preference)
3. Patient Bib
4. Bib Clip
5. Cotton Rolls and Gauze
6. Bite Block
7. Anesthetic Carpule
8. Mirror
9. Explorer
10. Cotton Pliers
11. Surgical Suction (disposable)
12. Monoject Syringe with Sterile Water
13. Periosteal Elevator
14. Currette
15. Bone File
16. Forcep

17. Forcep
18. Elevators
19. Wrist Blood Pressure Cuff
20. Post Op Pack for Patient (Gauze)
21. Topical Gel
22. Cotton Tip Applicator
23. Surgical Scissors
24. Suture
25. Hemostat
26. Damp Gauze
27. Minnesota Cheek Retractor

Sample Treatment Kit (Instruments)

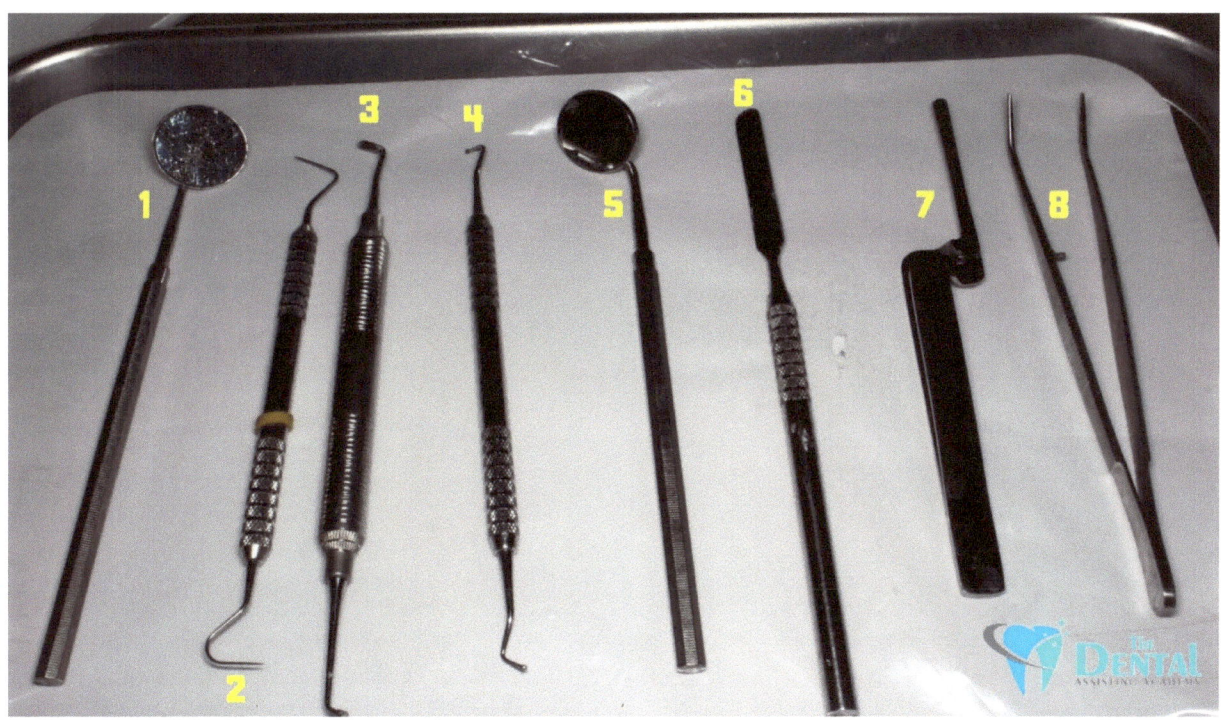

1. Mirror
2. Explorer
3. Flat Instrument/Ball Burnisher
4. Spoon Excavator
5. Mirror
6. Spatula
7. Articulating Paper Holder
8. Cotton Pliers

Oral Surgery Instruments (Review)

Forceps

a. 150 = Universal Upper
b. 151 = Universal Lower
c. 23 = Cowhorn Lower Molar
d. 88R = Upper Right Molar
e. 88L = Upper Left Molar
f. Beak = Anterior Root Tips
g. 69 = Anterior Premolar
h. Rontguers

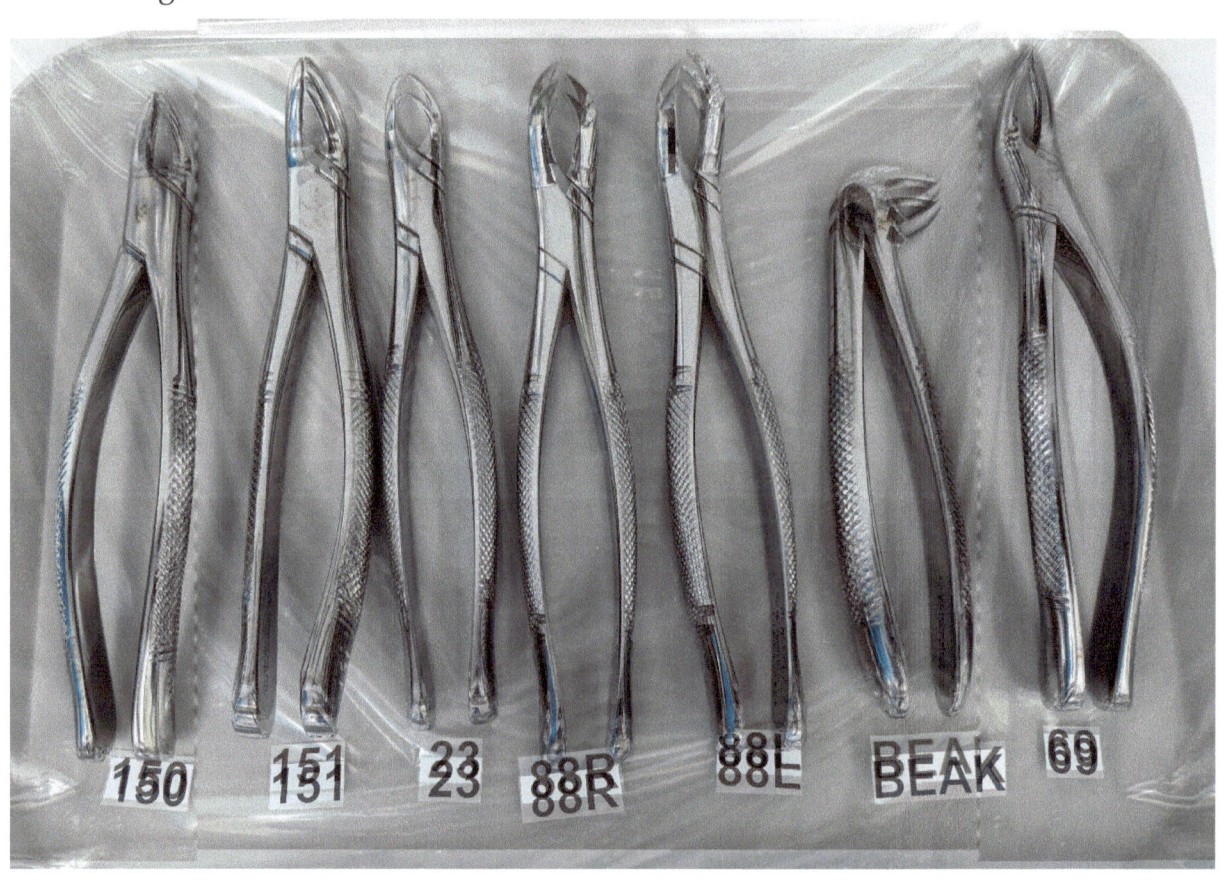

All Extraction Procedures Should Include:

   a. Straight Elevators
   b. East & West Elevators
   c. 3 Pack Periosteal (Molt Periosteal, Surgical Curette & Bone File)

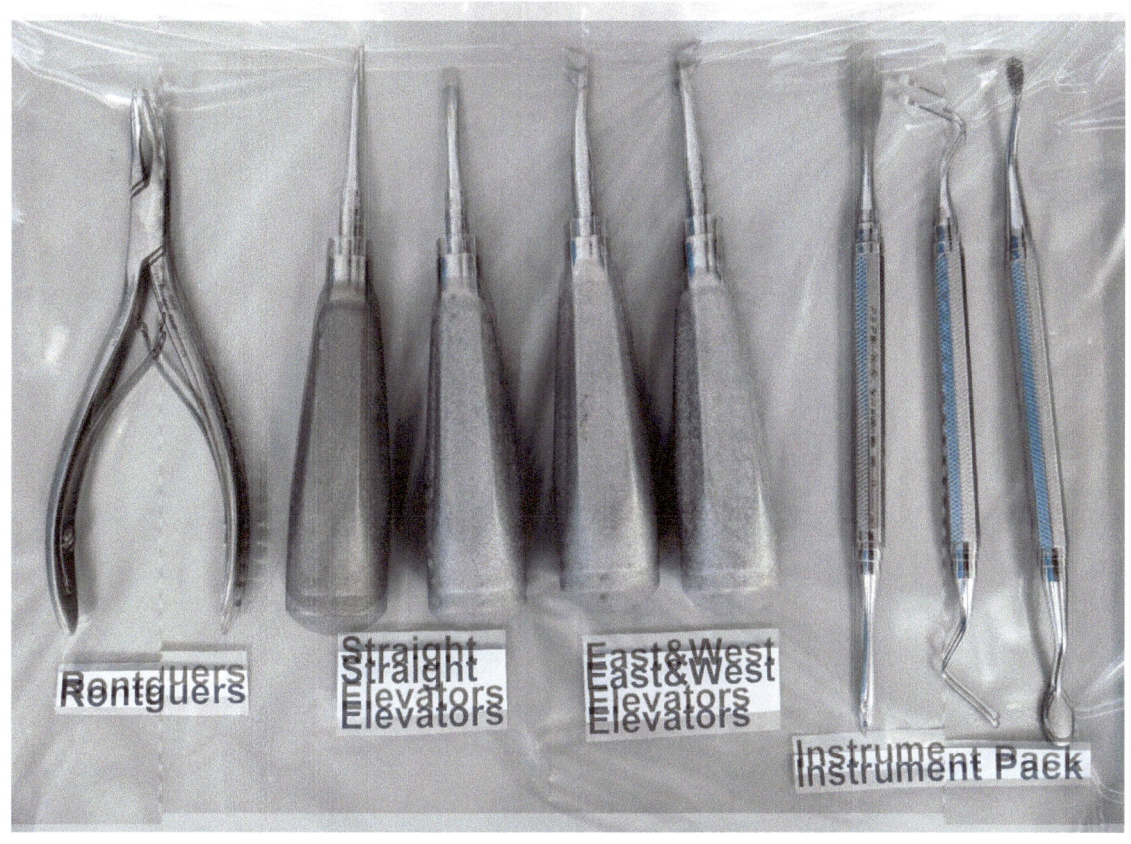

*All extraction instruments have identification numbers on the side.

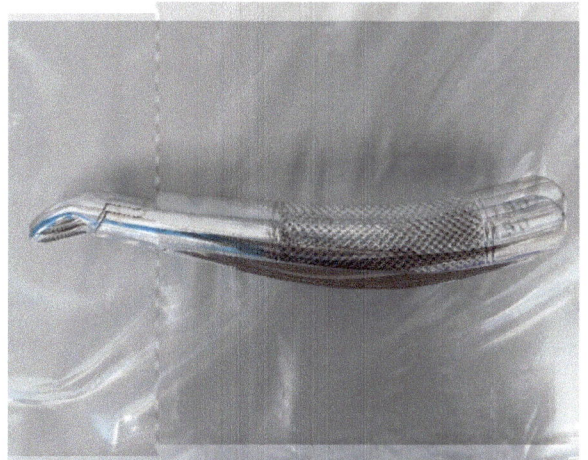
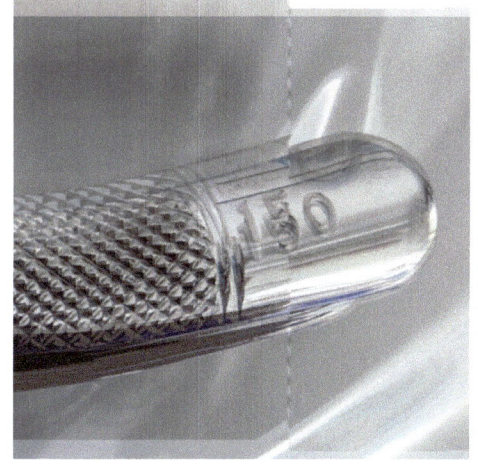

Ways To Advance Your Career

One of the quickest ways to advance you career is to STAND OUT. Standing out at work can have some great perks for you as a dental assistant. Whether you are a recent graduate or a seasoned professional, you can benefit from the tips listed below. Learn how to be the shining star of your dental team.

Build Great Patient Relationships

Building relationships with your patients is key to building a successful dental practice. Taking the time to get to know your patients and to build rapport makes you stand out as a super star dental assistant. It also makes the doctor happy to witness the patient feeling comfortable in the dental chair and interacting with the dental team.

Sell Other Dental Services

Once you build a great relationship with your patient, they will learn to trust you more and will be open to hearing your recommendations. This is a great opportunity to share your knowledge of products and additional services that may help them. This can be win for the practice as well as for you professionally.

Work Hard and Pick Up the Slack

Daily duties of a dental assistant will definitely keep you busy, but occasionally you will experience some down time. Be sure to keep busy during this time by helping your other team members with various task. If you are unsure, just ask who needs help. This may include assisting the hygienist, front office team or maybe the doctor. Either way, it is a great opportunity to learn more and grow in your new career. So, go beyond your daily duties and pick up the slack. You never know who notices your extra effort.

Consider Volunteering

Want to impress your boss? Spend some time volunteering. Not only will this help you find fulfillment with your new career, it also looks good on your resume. Doctors love to see that you spend some of your personal time helping others.

Continue Your Education

Never stop learning. You must complete a certain number of hours of continuing education each year to maintain your dental assistant license in most states. Find courses that interest you and can help you learn a new skill or technique. Make it fun. There are various courses available online.

Strive to be an extraordinary dental assistant. Go above and beyond for your patients, your doctor and your team. You never know when your efforts may be rewarded.

5 Ways to Comfort Your Patients

Dental anxiety is real. Studies show that 60% of people experience anxiety about visiting the dental office. As a dental assistant, you are in a great position to help your patients feel more comfortable in the dental chair. Here are 5 ways you can use to comfort your patients.

#1: Be welcoming to your patients

Greet your patients with a smile. Show them that you care and that you are there for them. Ask them how their day is going. Use small talk to ask them about family, hobbies or other interest. This will also help to distract the patient from thinking about their upcoming dental procedure. Your small gestures will not go unnoticed by your patients or your doctor.

#2: Help patients feel in control

Make a plan with the patient before the procedure starts. Let them know that they can raise their hand at anytime if they experience any pain or discomfort. Allowing the patient to feel in control, may help them to relax a bit more during the appointment.

#3: Use distractions

There are a few things you can do to help distract the patient from thinking about the dental procedure. Of course, talking to the patient helps. Soothing music can also help the patient feel relaxed. Other techniques like counting backwards or lifting their legs up and down can also help to distract the patient.

#4: Use education

Educate your patients. You learned a lot during dental assisting school. Share this information and knowledge with your patients. Help them understand the procedure they are about to receive. The more they understand, the less afraid they may feel. Be the expert!

#5: Always be professional

Your patients trust you and look to you for answers. Discuss your background and education with them so they can feel even more comfortable with you. You are more than qualified to this job. Do it well!

Using these tips can help you to create a comfortable environment for your patients where they can feel safe and cared for. Your patients will thank you for going the extra mile and your doctor will appreciate you helping to create competent and comfortable dental office.

Thank You

Thank you for purchasing and reading this book. It is my sincere hope that this book will help you in your new career as a dental assistant. I wish you the best! If you have more questions, connect with me using the various sources below.

Website

www.thedentalassistingacademy.com

Facebook

www.facebook.com/thedentalassistingacademy.com

YouTube

www.youtube.com/thedentalassistingacademy.com

Instagram

www.instagram.com/thedentalassistingacademy.com

About the Author

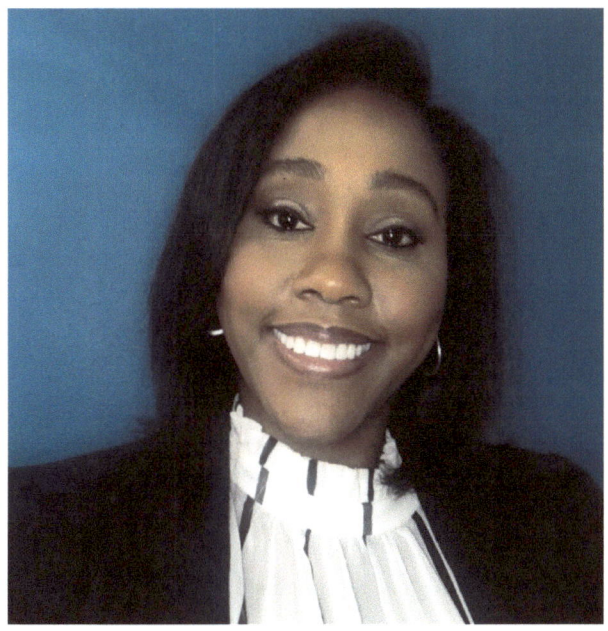

Dr. Kimberly Harper is a cosmetic and restorative dentist. She is passionate about helping others, and her professional life is centered around improving people's confidence by enhancing their smiles. One way she helps others is through her yearly mission trips to provide dental care to those in need in other countries.

Dr. Kimberly believes in developing a relationship with each of her patients to better listen to their needs and provide them with the best possible care. Along with her private dental practice, Dr. Kimberly is also the founder and dean of the Dental Assisting Academy, a twelve-week educational program that prepares students for certification as a dental assistant. She also has a YouTube channel, "Dr. Kimberly DDS," where she shares her knowledge of dentistry.

Dr. Kimberly can be contacted through her website, *www.thedentalassistingacademy.com*

www.ingramcontent.com/pod-product-compliance
Lightning Source LLC
Chambersburg PA
CBHW051944210526
45473CB00006B/2377